LITTLE BOOK OF
TAI CHI

LITTLE BOOK OF
TAI CHI

First published in the UK in 2013

www.demand-media.co.uk

Printed and bound in Europe.

ISBN 978-1-782811-83-1

The views in this book are those of the author but they are general views only and readers are urged to consult the relevant and qualified specialist for individual advice in particular situations.

In no way will Demand Media Limited or any persons associated with Demand Media be held responsible for any injuries or problems that may occur during the use of this book or the advise contained within. We recommend that you consult a doctor before embarking any exercise programme. This product is for informational purposes only and is not meant as medical advice. Performing exercise of all types can pose a risk, know your physical limits, we suggest you perform adequate warm up and cool downs before and after any exercise. If you experience any pain, discomfort, dizziness or become short of breath stop exercising immediately and consult your doctor

Contents

Introduction

Calm the mind, improve health, well-being, confidence and energise your body. The ancient spiritual art of Tai Chi does not require any overexertion, but, in fact, should be a totally enjoyable and profound experience.

Tai Chi is an internal Chinese martial art practised for both its defence training and its health benefits. It is also typically practised for a variety of other personal reasons: its hard and soft martial art technique, demonstration competitions and longevity. As a result, a multitude of training forms exist, both traditional and modern, which correspond to those aims. Some Tai Chi training forms are especially known for being practised at what most people categorise as slow movement. The term Tai Chi translates as 'supreme ultimate fist'.

The Little Book of Tai Chi introduces movements covering a form of Tai Chi created specifically to improve health that will help you to maintain or regain both your physical, emotional and mental health. By using controlled breathing and simple, flowing body movements, this can be achieved with as little as 20 minutes of Tai Chi a day.

You will be instructed on how to adjust yourself physically to do the

Tai Chi short form, but it is also important to prepare yourself mentally. Such instructions may be less familiar, as you are asked to 'hold the light ball' or to 'show your inner smile' for example. But with correct breathing and regular practice, feelings will come to life within you.

This book features Jason Chan who has practised Martial Arts, Tai Chi and Chi Kung since his childhood in Hong Kong. He now teaches Western students the arts of Infinite Chi Kung and Infinite Tai Chi and has transformed the lives of thousands of people all over the world. His programme Infinite Tai Chi for health with Jason Chan is also available on DVD to complement this volume.

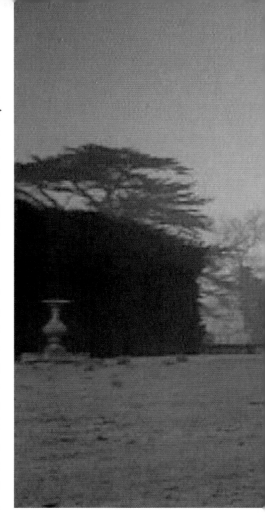

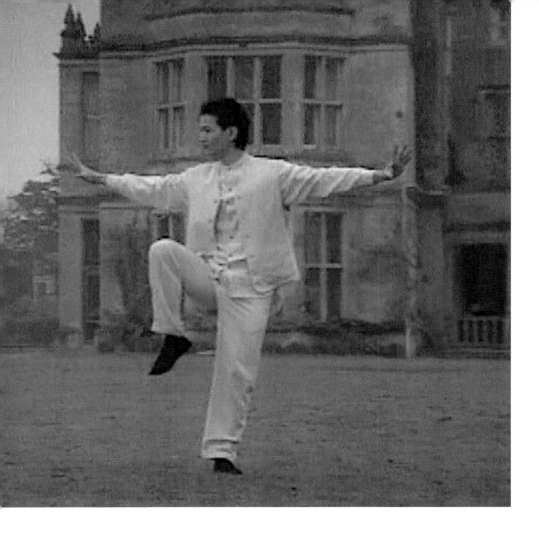

Chapter 1

Philosophy

The philosophy of Tai Chi begins with the belief that we are of the same universe as the natural elements and we have the same life force passing through us: Yin and Yang. How we manage our life force determines our physical and emotional well-being, and our mental peace of mind.

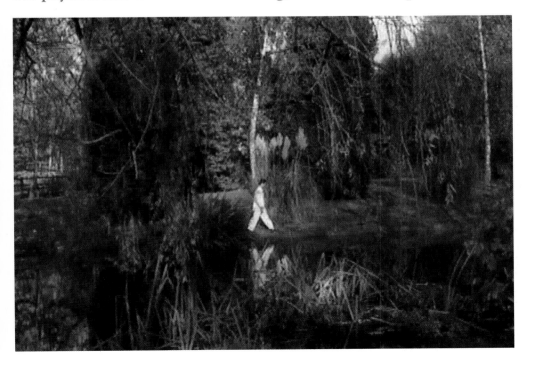

Chapter 2

Warming Up

Warming up for Tai Chi is done in a relaxed manner without strain, your mind open and clear. Stand with your feet firmly grounded, your toes pointing forward and your knees unlocked; allow your weight to sink as if you were sitting on a large balloon. This is known as the 'horse-riding' stance.

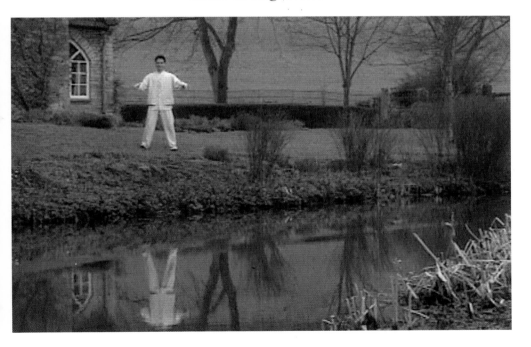

Now imagine that your abdomen is expanding outwards like an inflated balloon. Let it expand but remain well grounded. While breathing out, flatten your abdomen and gently pull the groin muscle up. Hold it and regulate your breathing.

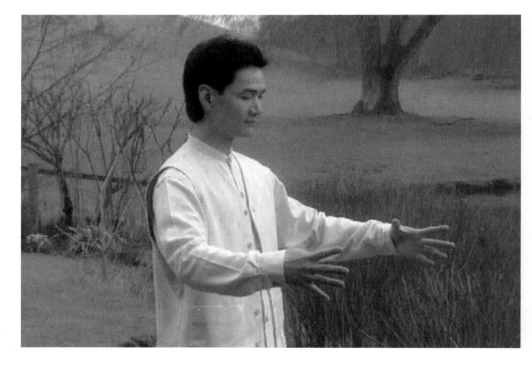

Now you are ready to raise the Chi. Put your palms down and relax your wrists, breathe in and raise your arms to shoulder level. Breathe out and sink them back down. Breathe in through your nose and out through your mouth as if blowing out a candle flame. Your tongue should rest against the roof of your mouth and your body should be relaxed. Repeat several times and get used to the rhythm of raising and sinking whilst remaining well grounded and breathing correctly.

Step 1

Step 2

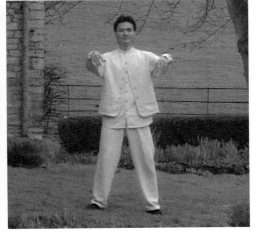 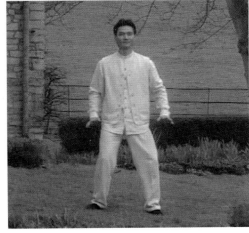

When you are ready to coordinate this exercise with your thoughts, breathe in, raise your palms and feel the lightness of the Chi. Breathe out, push down and feel its heaviness. Imagine you are pushing balloons down into water and feel the resistance as you push down and feel the lightness as you rise.

Step 1

Step 2

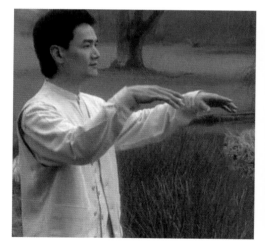

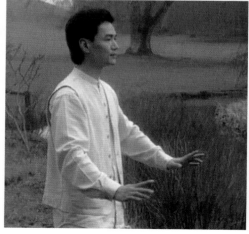

Now imagine that you are holding a ball of light about an inch below your naval at the Dan-Tien point.[1] There is no tension in your arms and your fingers are evenly spread.

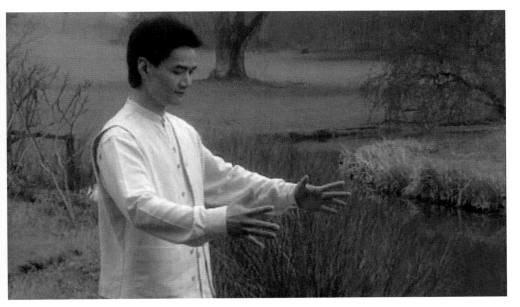

[1] A Daoist term referring to a centre of energy located midway between the navel and the pubic bone, inside the lower abdomen. The Dan-Tien is important as a balance focal point as the centre of balance in all people is located at a point that is at 40% of their height, which for nearly every person equates to their Dan-Tien point.

Regulate your breathing and relax your shoulders; if you become tense, remember your inner smile and relax. Allow the light ball to pulsate. With practice a force will be felt between your palms. This is the Chi energy. Breathe in and raise the light ball up through your head and back downwards breathing out. Imagine the light ball passing through your body, activating your Chi energy.

Step 1   Step 2

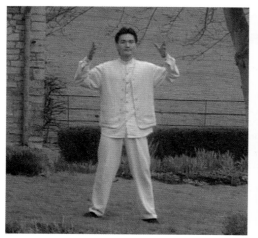 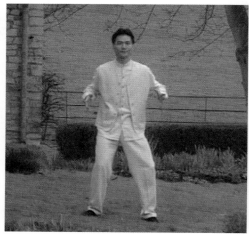

Then bring the light ball back to the Dan-Tien point. With your body relaxed, raise the light ball up above your crown centre and hold. Now lift your heels and hold for three seconds.

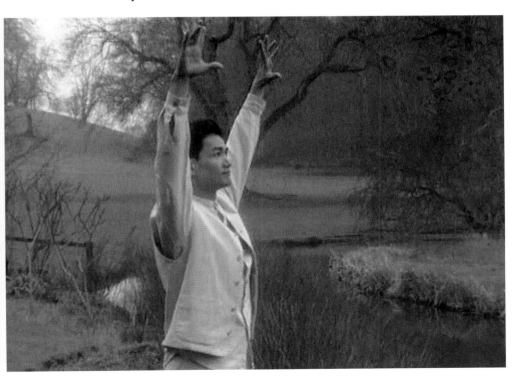

Bring your heels down and balance yourself. As you breathe out, bend your knees and bring the light ball down following it with your eyes and keeping your back straight with groin muscles tight. Hold for three seconds.

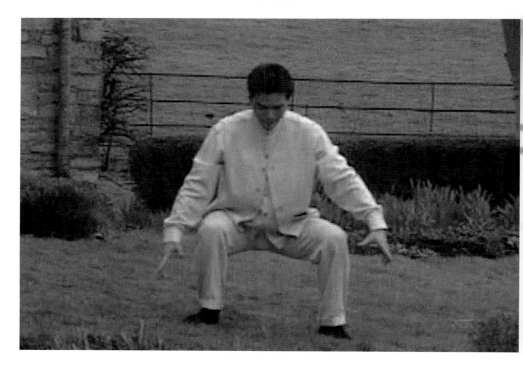

Breathe in, rising again. Think about your breathing and focus on the Chi energy in the light ball.

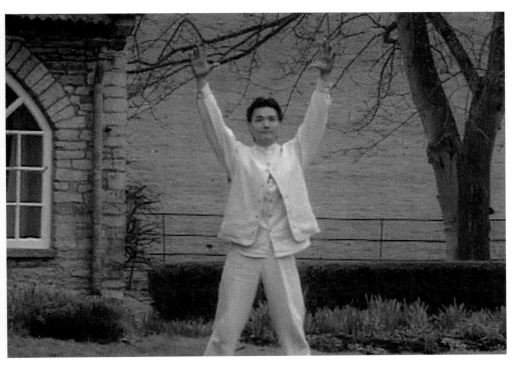

Focus on this sequence with the light ball for several minutes.

Next, ground yourself and extend your arms sideways as you breathe out.

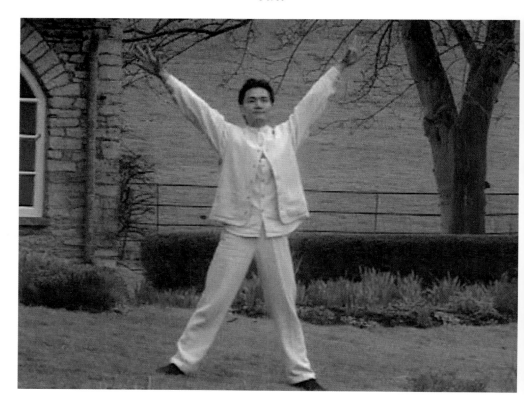

Bring your hands across the front of your body and breathe in.

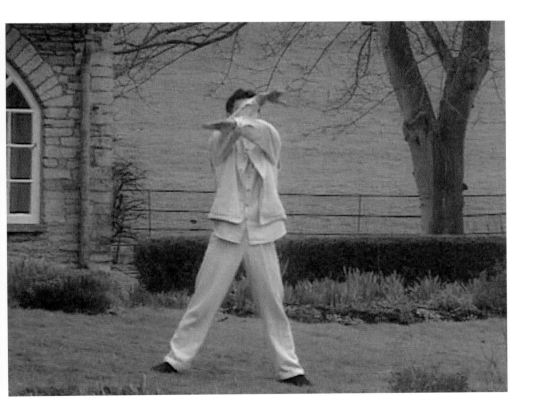

Spread your arms into a 'Y' shape and open your stance. Hold this for several seconds. With your fingers spread it pulls you upwards and at the same time the earth is pulling you downwards by your feet.

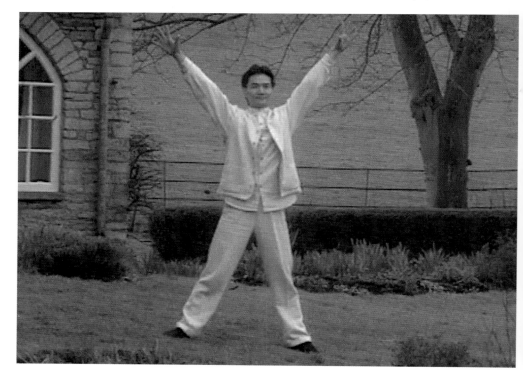

LITTLE BOOK OF **TAI CHI**

Then bring your hands back down and across your body and raise them up again. Repeat and stretch.

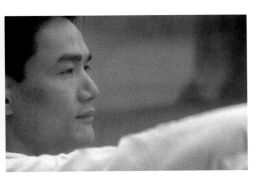

Step 1

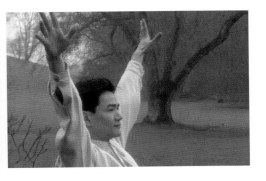

Step 2

Gently swing your arms to the left and right. Your eyes should follow your upper hand from side to side. Do several each side quite slowly, then speed up the swing from side to side.

Step 1

Step 2

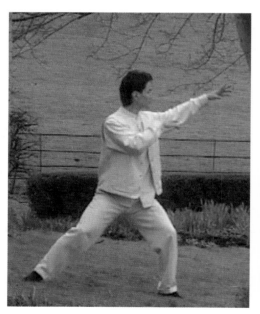

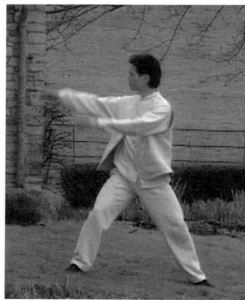

Then change direction: one arm swings towards the front, the other to the back. Use your waist to make the movement and your eyes follow the hand going backwards each time. Do several each side quite slowly, and then speed up the swing. Then slow down again with full control.

Step 1

Step 2

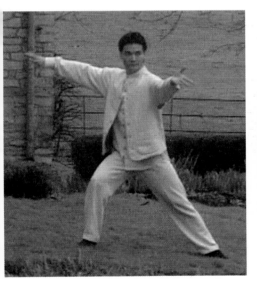 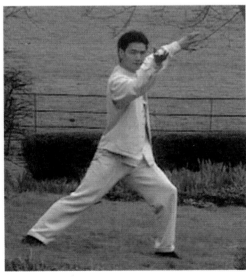

Repeat the sideways swinging movement.

Bring your arms to the Dan-Tien point.

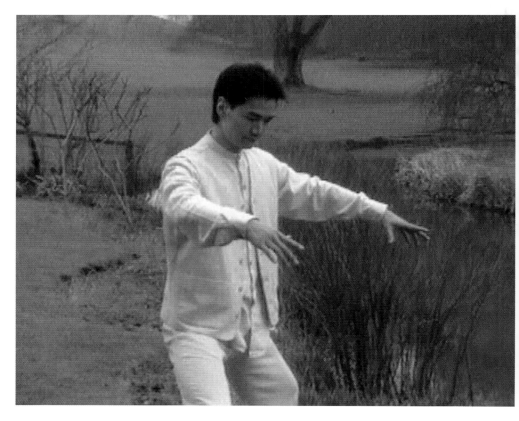

Resume the 'horse-riding' stance and regulate your breathing. Hold that position for several seconds. As you progress your stance and spine will become stronger and stronger. This will give you inner strength to perform the Tai Chi short form with full grace.

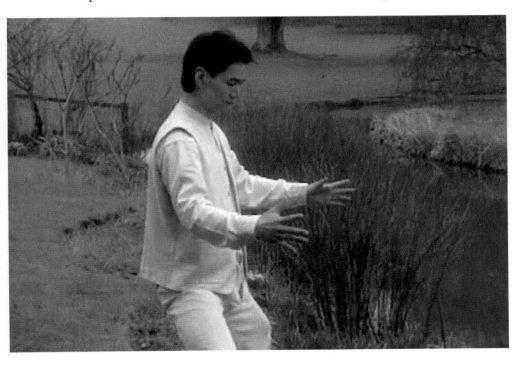

Individual joints must also be supple. First the wrists: with your feet shoulder width apart, raise your palms to chest level.

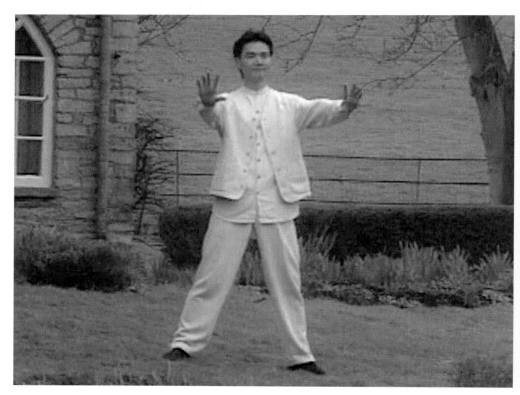

Turn your wrists gently on an inner circle nine times.

Step 1   Step 2   Step 3

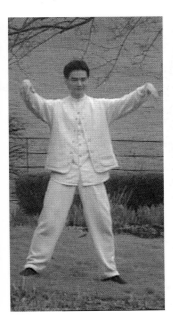
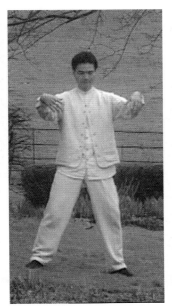
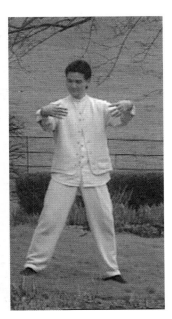

Then turn them in an outer circle nine times.

Step 1

Step 2

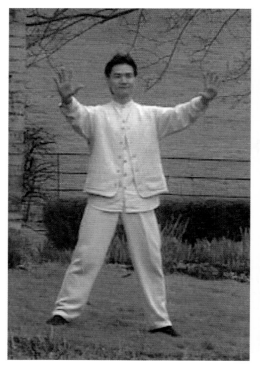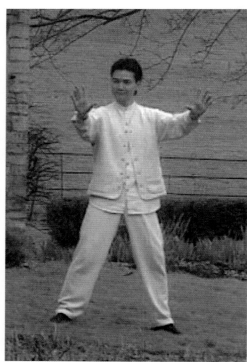

Now the fingers: clench your fists with your thumbs folded inside.

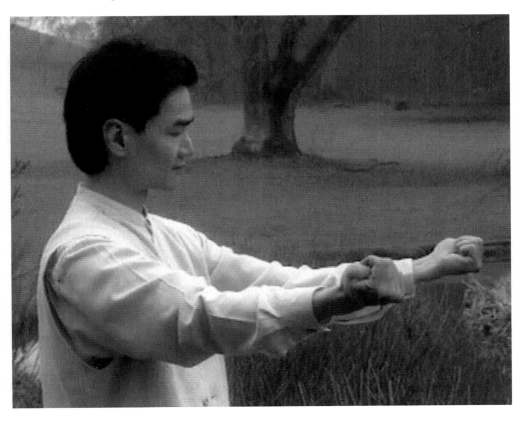

Deliberately flick the fingers outwards some eighteen to thirty-six times. Think about your stance and regular breathing.

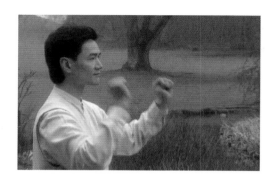

Step 1

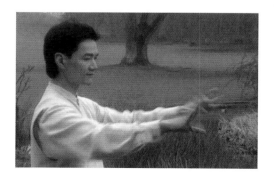

Step 2

The final part of the warm-up is to stretch your body and legs. Spread your feet wide apart and use your right fingers to touch your left toes and your left fingers to touch your right toes. Your head and spine should be alined. Continue the exercise for a minute or so.

Step 1   Step 2

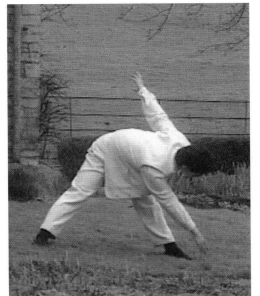 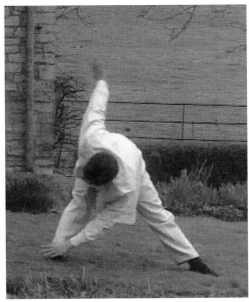

Re-centre yourself and try to use your palms to touch the ground and let them support part of your body weight.

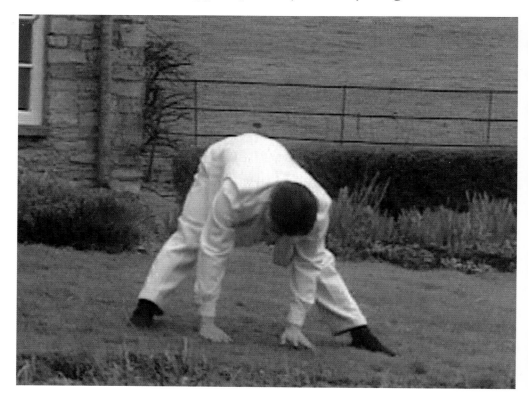

Bend your right knee and straighten your left leg and stretch. Now move across bending the left knee and straightening the right leg. Do this six times on each side.

Step 1

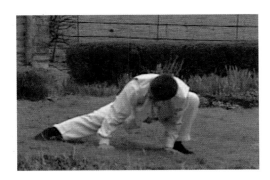

Step 2

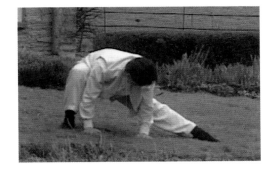

Slowly and carefully raise yourself to an upright position. Imagine there is someone else holding you under your armpits gently pulling you upright; allow your whole body to relax.

Step 1

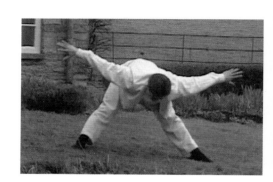

Step 2

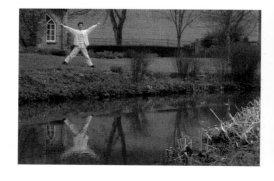

Chapter 3

Breathing

Regulated breathing is one of the foundations of Tai Chi.

Stand with your feet apart and centre yourself.

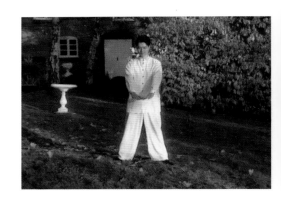

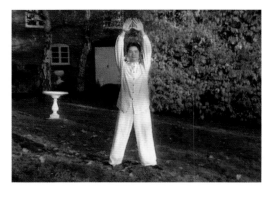

Bring your two hands together and as you raise your hands slowly upwards, breathe in the Chi. Focus on this movement.

As your hands divide over your head, consciously bring down the Chi energy to envelop your whole body in an oval shape.

Step 1

Step 2

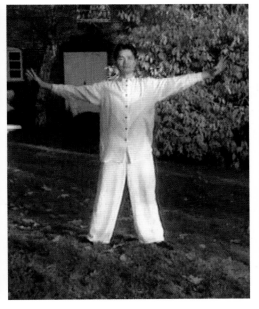

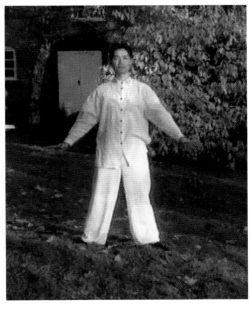

Breathe in through the Dan–Tien point and pull your abdomen up slowly, expand your chest and fill your lungs with fresh air; palms facing upwards to the sun, breathe in the essence of life itself through your whole being, through your fingertips. Repeat twice.

Step 1

Step 2

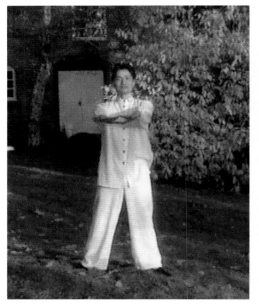 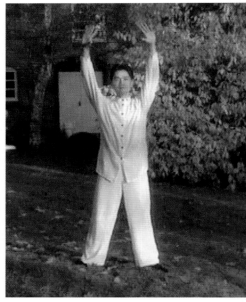

Bring both hands down to the side of your body, slowly breathe in and bring your palms up again, towards the centre of the chest.

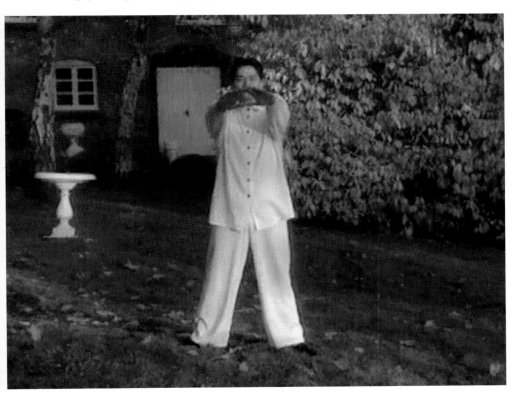

Chapter 4

Simple Movements

To help an individual maintain and regulate a state of balance, a series of simple movements can be performed.

Balanced Walking

Do not use your muscle strength, use the mind and the flow of your Chi. Balanced walking is a slow movement with the mind focused on the fullness of your weight on the one side and the lightness on the other, and the slow transfer of weight as you move forward. As you walk, imagine that there is a thread of light from heaven anchored on top of your head pulling you up. Breathe easily and use your mind's eye to focus on the Dan–Tien point to achieve balance.

Step 1

Step 2

Step 3

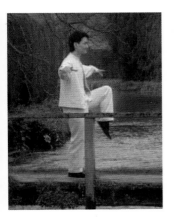
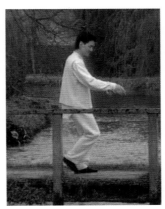
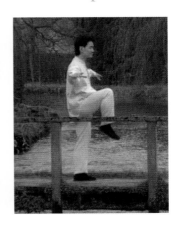

Standing Like A Tree

Spread your legs apart and adopt the 'horse-riding' stance, feet firmly routed to the ground with your body as the trunk and your hands as the two main branches.

Hold for several seconds.

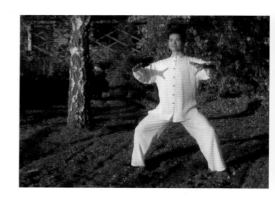

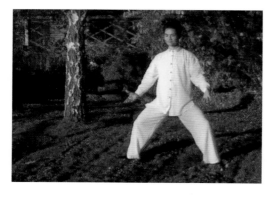

Breathe out as you bring your hands down and shake off the tension in your shoulders.

Breathe in and raise them back up again.

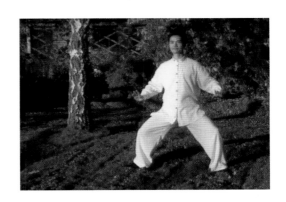

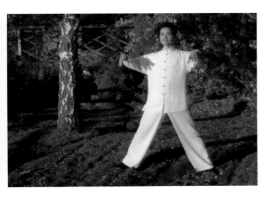

Bring back the elbows and breathe out as your hands go down and feel the sinking effect.

Waving Hands Like The Clouds

By caressing the air and feeling the lightness, you will bring out your inner smile. Our muscles have limitations, but the Chi has no limitations. The movements of the heavenly bodies and the natural elements are circular; these are the important rhythms of life.

Step 1   Step 2   Step 3

 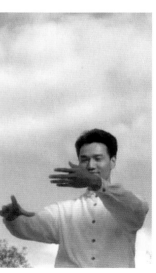 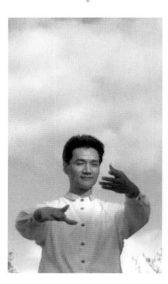

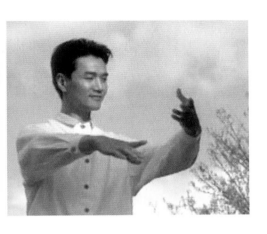

Step 4

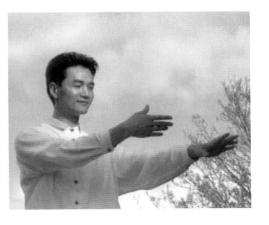

Step 5

Chapter 5

Five Elemental Movements

There are five elemental movements that allow you to control your Chi energy in a way that rebalances the ups and downs and stresses and strains of day-to-day life.

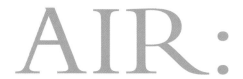

AIR:

to calm yourself and be conscious of life. Combine your breathing with the rhythm of the movements shown in the pictures. Breathe in through your nose as you expand yourself, and then breathe out through your mouth slowly.

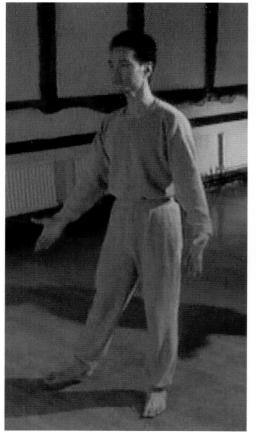
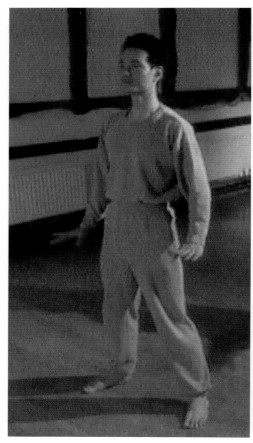

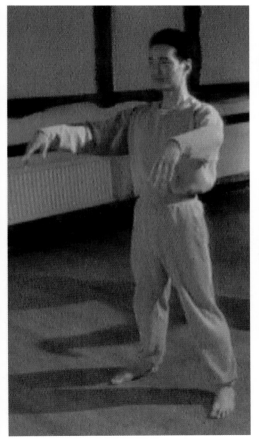
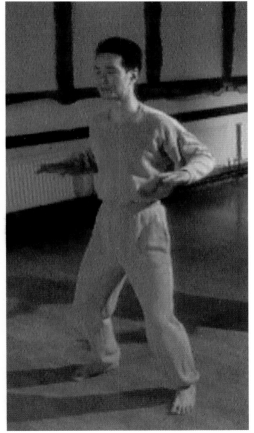

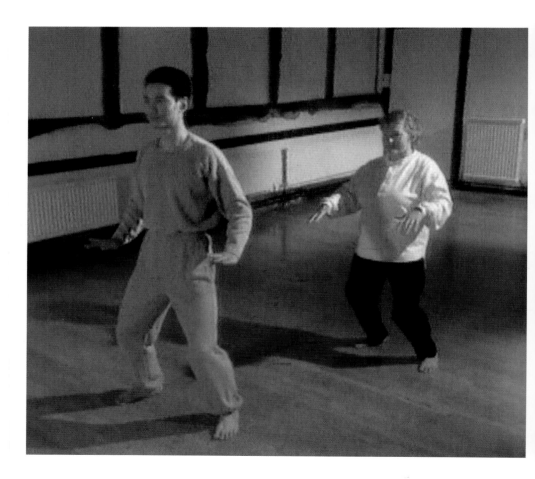

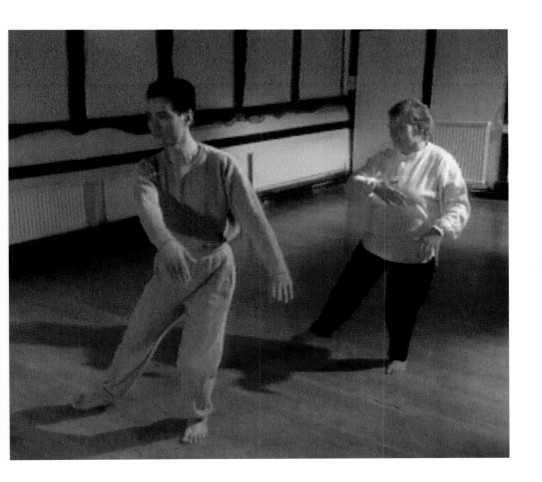

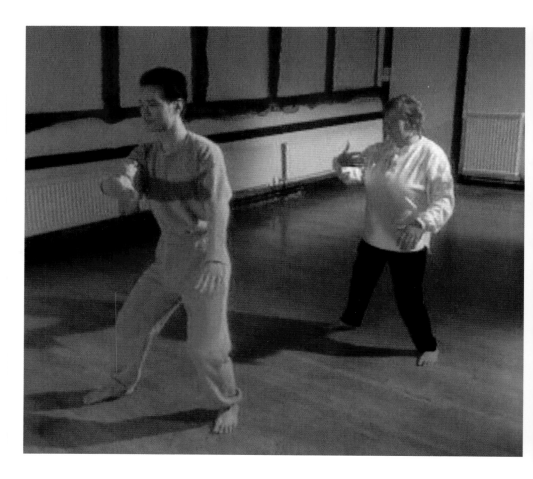

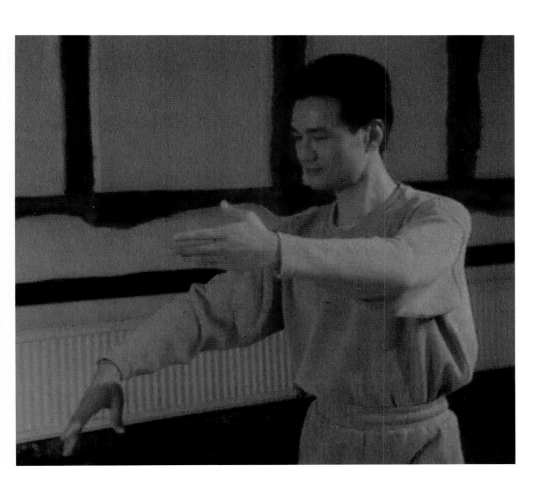

EARTH:

to be still; rooted like a tree. Adopt the 'horse–riding' stance, centre yourself and breathe in through the abdomen.

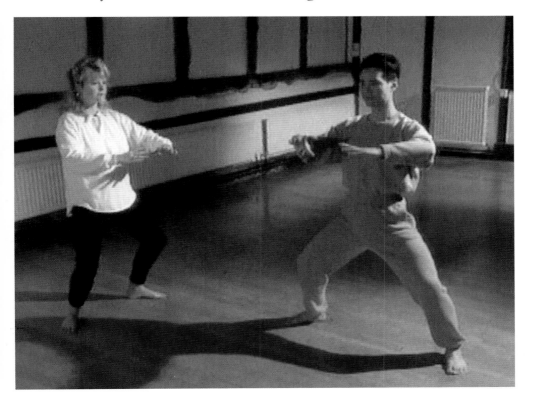

As you breathe in extend your arms.

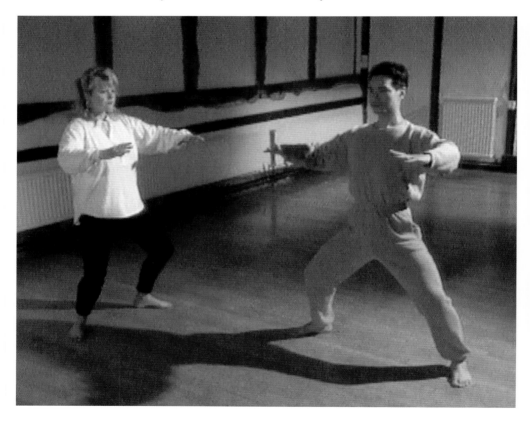

As you breathe out, contract and feel yourself sinking down.

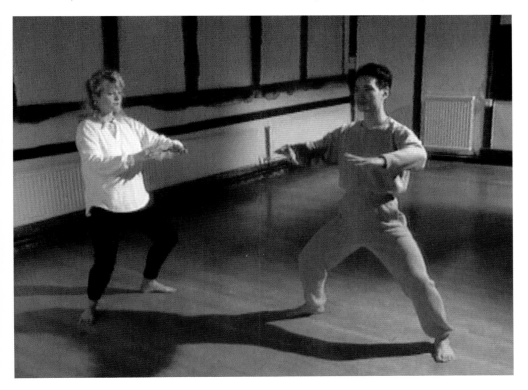

Repeat this controlled and gentle movement several times.

Standing with your feet together, move into the 'horse-riding' stance and breathe in.

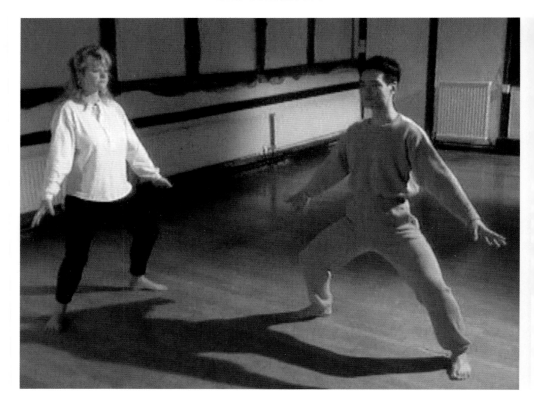

Slowly pull the Chi into your abdomen with your hands.

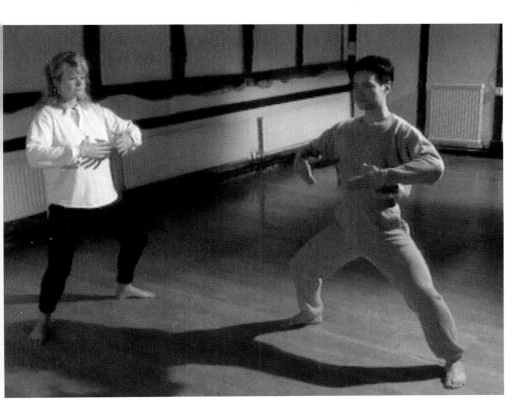

Breathe out and bring the hands to the side of your body but sink down.

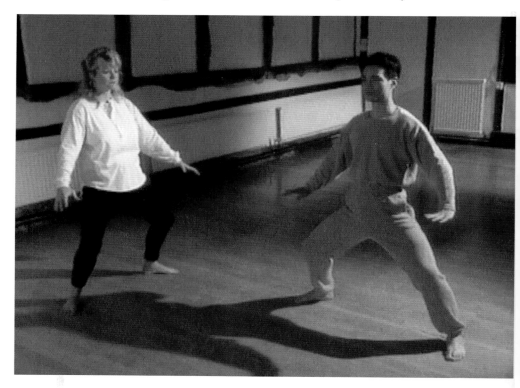

Repeat this controlled and gentle movement several times.

Standing with your feet together, move into the 'horse-riding' stance and breathe in. Drop the hands to the Dan-Tien point then raise them and clench your fists.

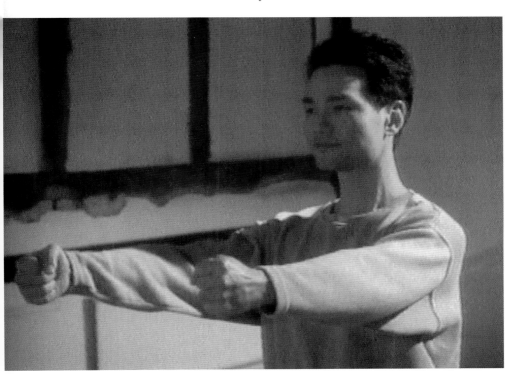

Pull them out and breathe in at the same time, relaxing your shoulders.

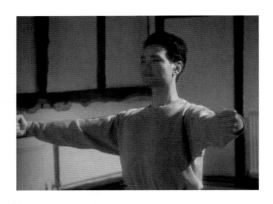

Step 1

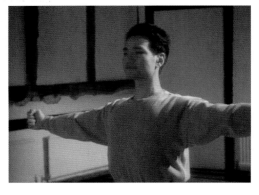

Step 2

Drop the hands whilst slowly breathing out.

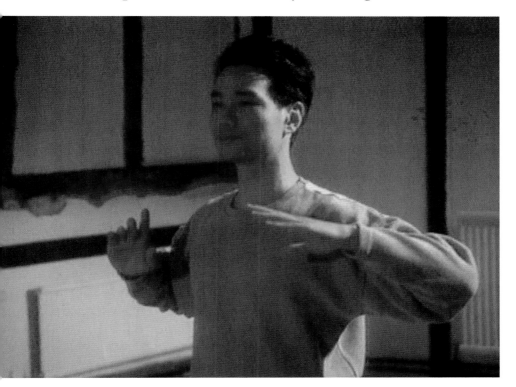

Repeat this controlled and gentle movement several times.

FIRE:

to raise vitality to face the day. Follow the sweeping arm movements shown in the pictures and focus on the outward sweep of your palms. Breathe in as you move upward; breathe out as you return. Try to remain centred. The body moves gracefully, without effort and without force.

Repeat this controlled and gentle movement several times.

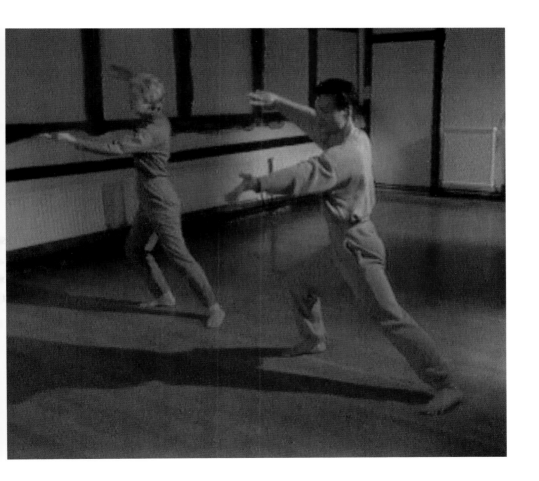

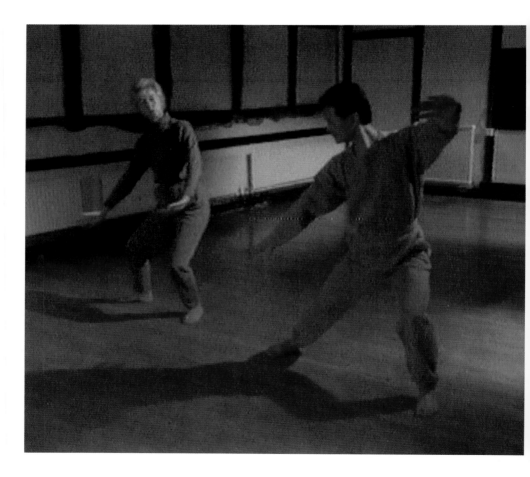

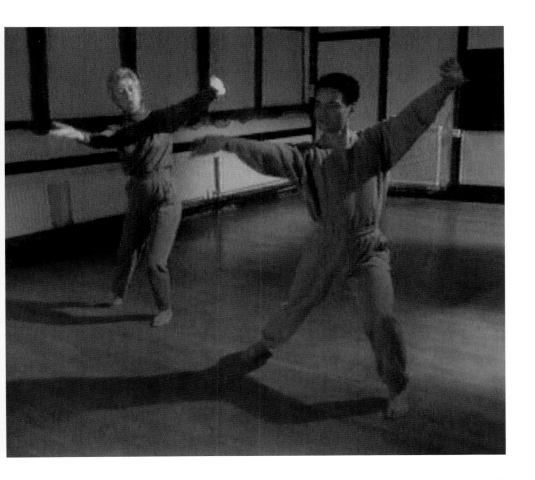

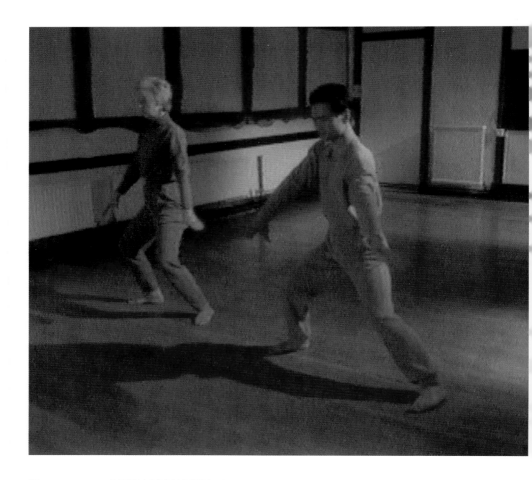

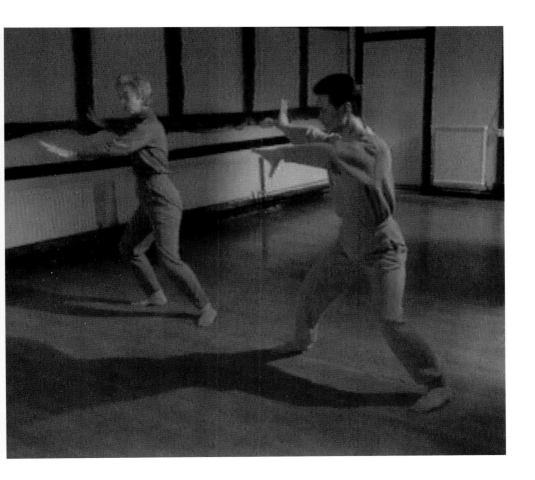

WATER:

to allow your feelings to flow out. Think of the ripples made by a falling leaf in a still pond. Slowly spread outwards in a gentle, circular rhythm. Imagine your middle fingers touching the surface of the water. Trace the ripples as they gently fade outwards to stillness.

Repeat this controlled and gentle movement several times.

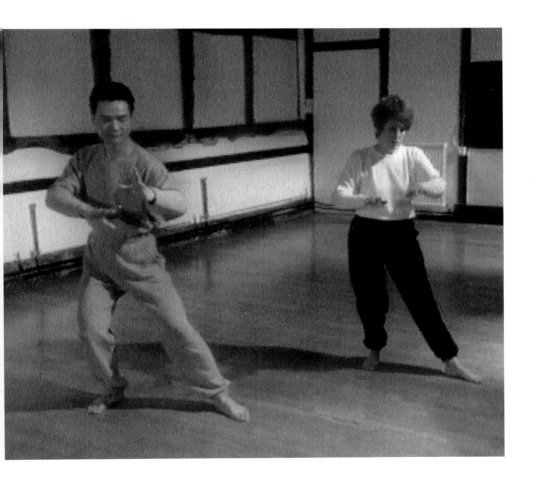

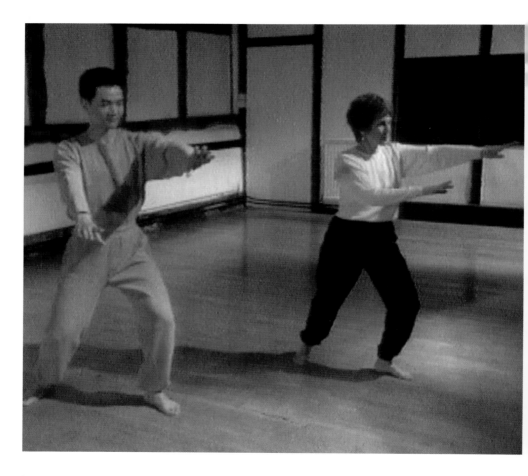

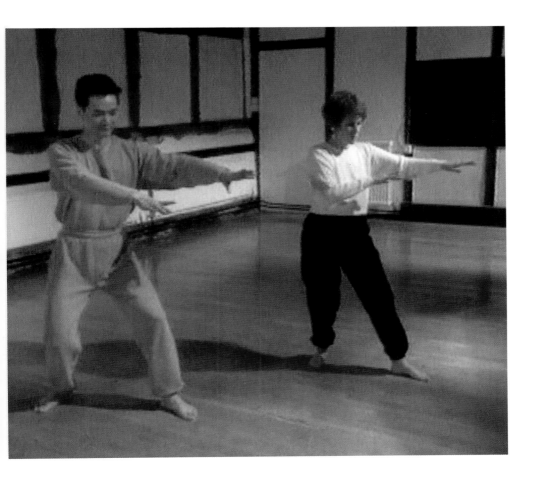

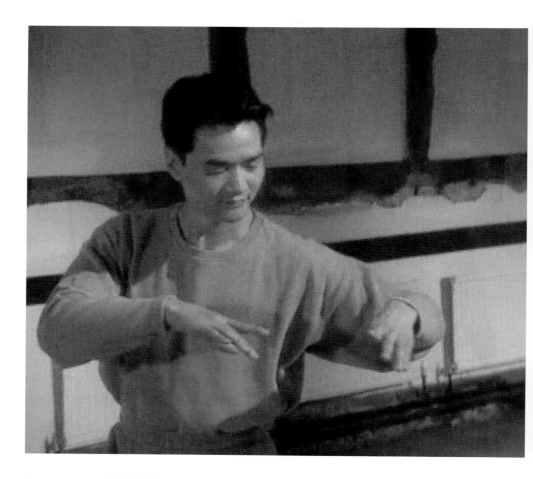

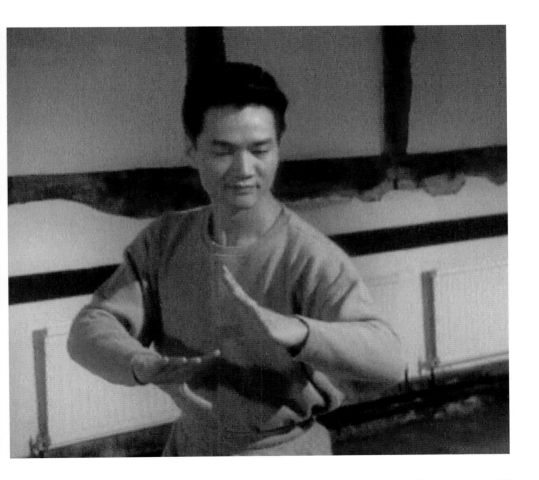

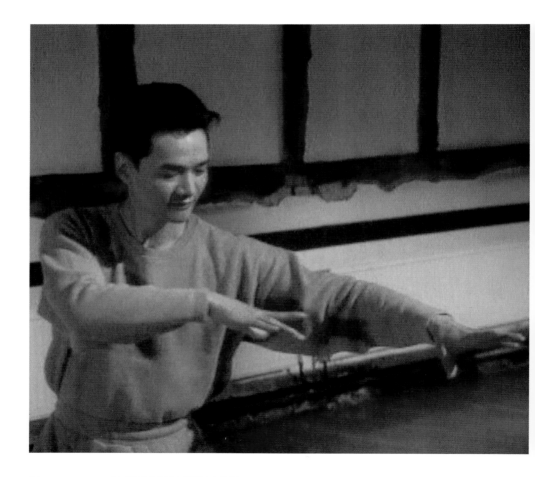

Then surge downwards and feel the unceasing forward motion, full flowing and free. Breathe out on the downward movement; let your feelings flow out.

Step 1

Step 2

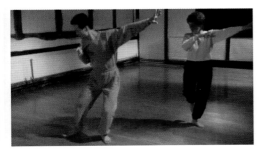

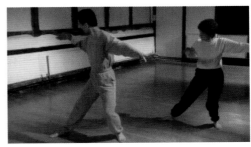

Step 3

Step 4

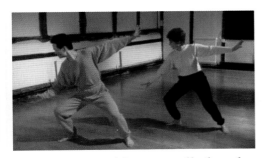

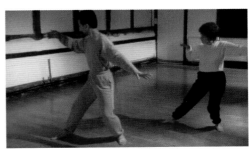

Repeat this controlled and gentle movement several times.

BALANCE:

through pushing hands. Stand comfortably and gently touch together the backs of your wrists. Move your right hand in an anti-clockwise circular motion as you move backwards and forwards. In your heart, feel a welcome for your partner and express this appreciation in your circular movement.

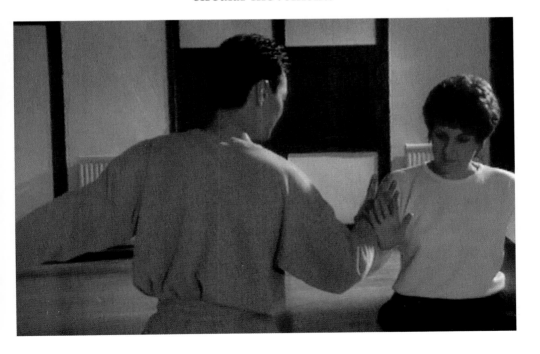

Focus on your breathing and calm your thoughts. Your movement will become smooth and relaxed, bringing added peace of mind and harmony to you both.

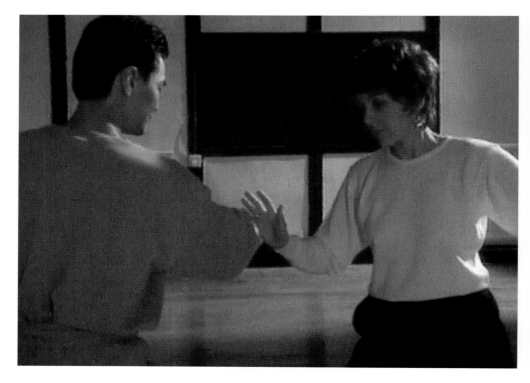

Done properly this exercise releases rigidity of the hips and shoulders. When you change to your left hand, remember the circular motion becomes a clockwise movement.

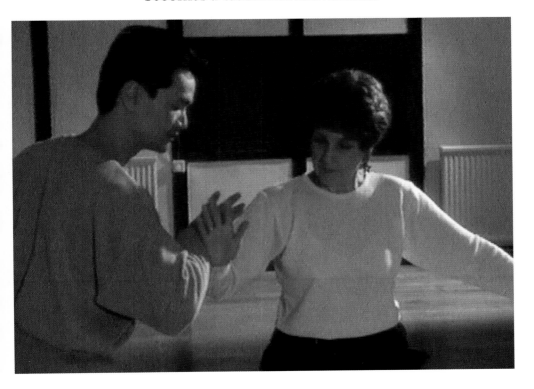

Practising Tai Chi for ten minutes a day leaves students feeling relaxed, alert and full of energy. The short form transforms the energy within us, allowing our Chi to flow freely and helping to relieve many conditions. You can regain the power to tell your body how it feels. You will be able to cope with stress and relieve anxiety and sleeplessness.

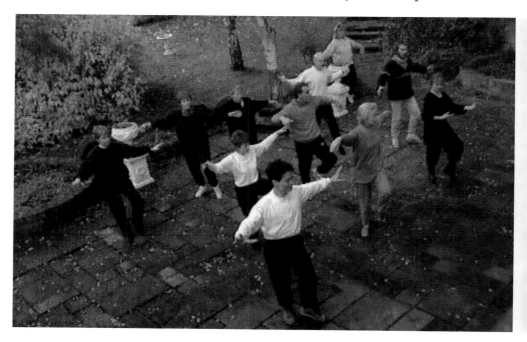

Tai Chi exercise also gives a sense of freedom through the movements that will help to relieve joint pain, back pain, and migraines. By discovering your inner beauty, not only will your overall health improve, but so will your personal self esteem.

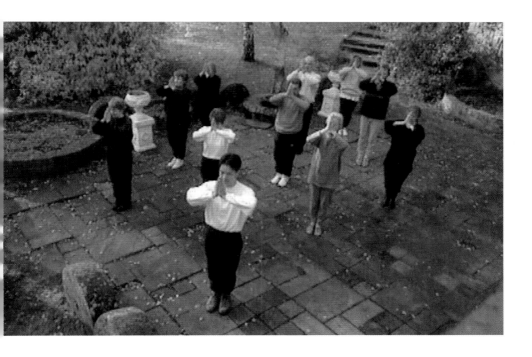

Chapter 6

Warm Down

At the end of Tai Chi exercise, it is just as important to warm down as it was to warm up.

Stand with your feet apart, soft knees and with your fingers pointing up. Breathe in through your nose and raise your arms.

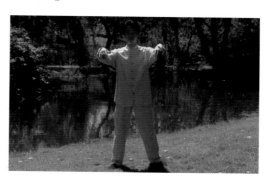

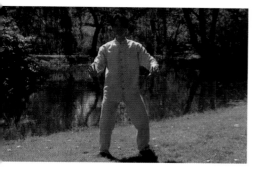

Breathe out through your mouth and sink down.

Repeat five times.

Swing your body from side to side rotating from the hips in a very relaxed and gentle manner. Repeat ten times.

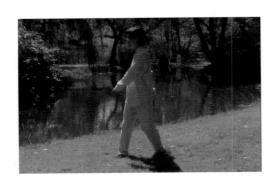

Step 1

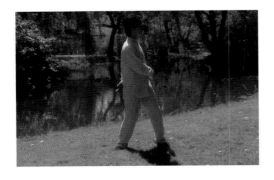

Step 2

Gradually extend your arms, rising. Repeat ten times.

Step 1

Step 2

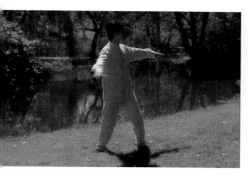

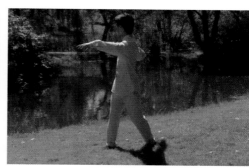

imagine that you are holding a light ball between your palms, gradually swinging back to the centre.

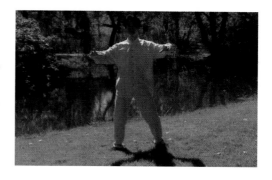

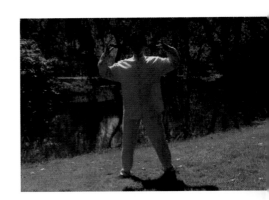

Holding the light ball, breathe in and bring the light ball up and in towards you.

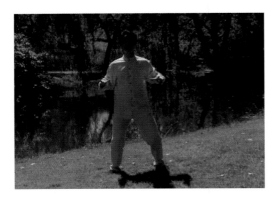

Breathe out slowly and lower the light ball, sinking.

Repeat five times.

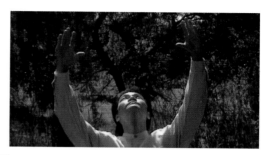

Breathe in, rising upwards and bring the light ball above your head.

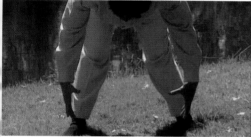

Breathing slowly out, bring the light ball all the way down, staying very relaxed.

Repeat five times and bring the ball back to the centre.

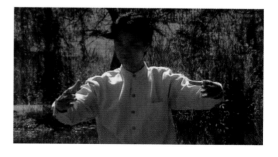

Breathe in and expand the light ball.

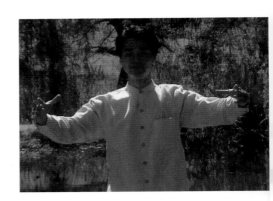

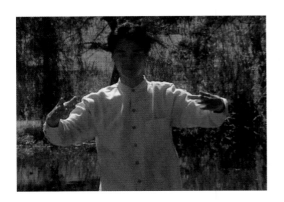

Breathe out and contract the light ball.

Repeat five times.

Put your hands down and your feet together, breathing in, raise your arms.

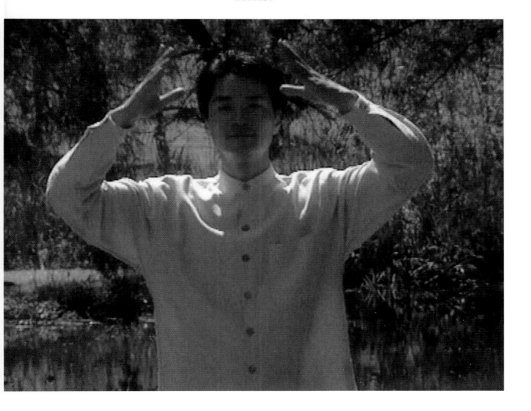

Breathing out, bring them gently down again.

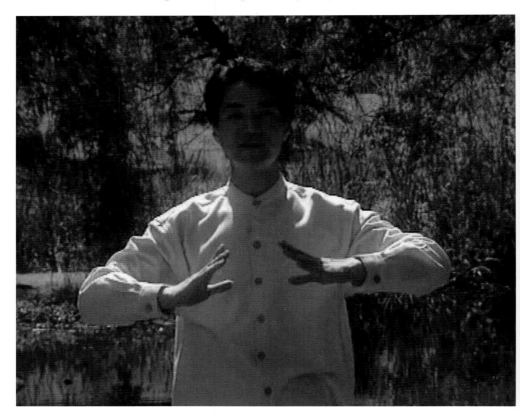

First swing your arms gently, and then introduce kicking your legs and enjoy your day!

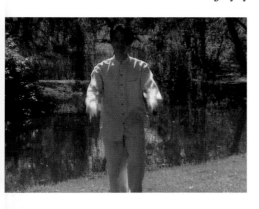

Step 1

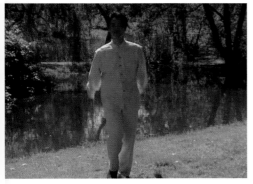

Step 2

Design and artwork by Scott Giarnese

Published by Demand Media Limited

Publishers Jason Fenwick & Jules Gammond

Written by Michelle Brachet